Giving BIRTH TO HIV

JOYFUL SOUL

The sale of this book without its cover is unauthorized. If you purchased this book without a cover, you should be aware that it was reported to the publisher as "unsold and destroyed". Neither the author nor the publisher has received payment for the sale of this "stripped book".

Copyright © 2017 Joyful Soul

Editor Cee Elle Reid

All rights reserved.

Large Print.

ISBN: 1979820805
ISBN-13: 978-1979820806

DEDICATION

In memory of my husband.

May you rest blessed knowing the love we shared.

CONTENTS

	Acknowledgments	i
1	Surprise	1
2	Confession	Pg 4
3	Karma	Pg 7
4	Forgiveness	Pg 10
5	Second Proposal	Pg 13
6	Wedding	Pg 16
7	Baby Fever	Pg 18
8	Affair	Pg 24
9	Reception	Pg 26
10	Home Sweet, Home	Pg 31
11	Morning Sickness	Pg 34
12	New Year's Resolution	Pg 37
13	The Fall	Pg 39
14	Diagnosis and Devotion	Pg 42
	Stay Current NAM Article	Pg 45

ACKNOWLEDGMENTS

My Dad, for allowing me to be me and helping me to understand the power of forgiveness.

VF and KB, for seeing a side of me which I couldn't see when we began this growing journey.

My children, for being patient with my mothering and growing through this process together.

1 SURPRISE

I felt like I gave birth to death. April 11, 2013, I woke up to the man I had been loving in secret. He didn't know me and I had not known him, yet the passion to be with him came more natural than any one-night stand. He had a part of my soul that I couldn't turn my back on. Waking up next to him gave life to my purpose; it felt good not to be judged and just live in the moment.

Tony and I shared it all, yet the

passion behind his eyes held some deep pain. When you love a soul that had experienced life three decades preceding your birth, it's natural to understand he has been through some things. It didn't matter because, in every moment, he proved who he wanted to be to me.

Today was the day after I turned twenty-seven years old. Seemed like another day of him and I living in the moment and not caring about the judgments faced by us; until he wanted to take me to "dinner." I'm no stranger to food; he knew that because, for two years, he has been my personal chef.

The most important thing about our bond is the love he shared with Jacob. This is the reason he won my heart. Three months earlier when he asked me to marry him, it was easy to say yes. We are both getting ready for our date and I asked, "Are we taking Jacob?" He responded sternly, "No, he is staying with your mom but I will stop by to give him some money." I knew loving this man was so right; I didn't have to beg him to father my son.

The arrival to my mom and stepdad's house was nothing out of the ordinary at first, until I saw a banner that read, "Happy Birthday, Shannon," with a picture of Jacob and I. I looked at everyone as I got closer and realized he kept a secret from me and was smiling with everyone else. I palmed my face in disbelief.

When I snapped out of my shocked state, I was called to the attention of my mother with her hand waving; motioning me in her direction. She was sitting next to one of her talking buddies, Ms. G, there was no telling where their conversation was going.

Ms. G says, "Is that TJ?"

I had never referred to Tony as TJ, but I knew everyone else did, for some reason he didn't want me calling him TJ.

I proceeded to answer her but my defense for my love kicked in, so I replied, "Yes, that's him. Why?"

"That mother f****r has HIV!" she replied.

2 CONFESSION

My heart dropped. I was in shock and tears feeling like sharp blood drops filled my eyes. I never felt so humiliated in my life. I thought waiting to know each other on that level was something to be valued and was a decision we made together. At the moment, it only felt like a method to keep me blindfolded.

I reached for his hand and asked him to sit in the car with me. I needed him to help me understand how he knows Ms. G and why she would say that about him.

"That b***h don't know me," he said.

At that point, I could remember asking myself, "Why isn't he denying this painful accusation so we can move on?"

We were back in the car, away from the world, yet the whispering at the party continued on. Finally, I was safe with him, where I had been for two strong years.

"Tony, I need the truth, what is this woman talking about?" I had to break the tension by asking him that question.

Again he replied, "that b***h don't know me."

This time my aggression towards his manipulation grew and I begin to get frustrated. "Stop with the bull and tell me the truth!"

"What do you want to know?" he asked.

The confirmation she was right, became clearer with his response. Although the heaviness of this tragic news put me in total confusion, my love for him became covered with the hate I thought I was supposed to have; because it's what others expected. I gave him his ring back.

"How long have you known?" I asked as tears of disappointment flowed down my face.

The magnitude of how long he kept this from me became an immediate worry.

Who is going to love me now? Who is going to protect my son from this hurt, I feel? What will he feel when he figures out that it's over between the two of us?

While I cried Tony spoke in the softest tone, "I wanted to tell you for so long but as I got to know you, I fell in love with you and didn't want to lose that feeling. I have been dealing with HIV for about twenty-two years and I have it under control; I have never infected anyone."

I left the car and went running in my mom's arms. This was my heaven as a child. She gave my soul a steady stream of balance and healing when I needed it most. Many times my mother and I never saw eye to eye, however, this deception was something that brought us together as time passed.

The growing feeling of abandonment and weakness would not escape from me. I was in love with a man who didn't trust me enough to let me choose if I wanted to conceive this secret. We had engaged in conceiving a life together; now I had to explore the dynamics of this miscarriage. He tore out the core of my love, the trust I thought we shared.

Moving forward was hard with our current living situation. The most complicated thing about loving a man who broke my heart was living in the suite below him and his daughter. Having to see him in passing the next few days became stressful. My heart yearned for the companionship. I was not ready to give up.

3 KARMA

I was watching a movie late one night and someone knocked on the door. No one came to my house without calling; it was an unspoken rule. I tried to ignore the knocking, then my phone rang; it was Tony's daughter, Tamika.

"Hello," The curiosity was heavy in my voice when I answered the phone.

"Hey, Shan. I need to talk to you, can you open the door?" she sobbed.

As I hung up the phone and answered the door, I asked her what was wrong. "I feel so horrible," she said.

"Why?" I asked.

"When you asked me why I didn't tell you that my father was HIV positive and I said it wasn't my place," her voice broke through the sobbing, "well I got the news I am HIV positive also!"

"It's going to be okay," I reassured her. "If your dad can live a healthy life, then you can too."

We talked more about how much will be ahead for her and her family. The days following were kind of a blur. I couldn't help feeling like karma gave her exactly what she deserved, yet no one deserves this type of betrayal.

The mixed emotions I was feeling were so heavy I had to share them with someone. I called the last person on earth who was worthy of my friendship or even conversation. As the phone rang I second-guessed the reason I was breathing life back into this situation.

"Hey, you have reached the voicemail of TJ—"

I began to get lost in my thoughts and started to think about situations that could have led to Tamika's current diagnosis. I can remember when they moved in above me. There was a revolving door of men around her sons which was not a good look.

The guys she attracted were the most disrespectful, boundary crossing, uneducated black boys I had ever seen. I make this statement due to the smoking of marijuana around my door and them leaving beer cans and cigarette ends in the parking lot. I had a good idea as to where she contracted the condition.

The recent men she had sex with were all negative: her baby daddy, her ex, and her current boyfriend. There was this guy she became re-acquainted with from Winston-Salem who I fussed with Tony about because he took the guy back to Winston-Salem every weekend.

He just gave me a bad vibe and I didn't want him around my son. We were living in High Point at the time. In the back of my head, I am still convinced it was him; however, I never knew his name.

4 FORGIVENESS

I hung up the phone and thought about inviting someone over to help me pass the time but before I could finish my thought Tony was knocking on the door. I knew it was him due to the heaviness of the knock. Before I could get out of bed he was walking in my room. I froze.

In the midst of everything that happened, I never took my key back. I realized in that moment he respected my space while still having complete access to me. The sight of him walking into the room, looking good and smelling like the Polo Black I love so much, took my mind back to the place we were two weeks ago; before the storm.

"You called me baby?" His voice was deep and sexy. I tried not to give him any indication I needed him or help me sort through my thoughts.

"Yeah, I called. You didn't have to come down here and where are you going dressed up?" There was no way he was going out tonight; not on my watch. One thing that would always make him stay was Jacob.

"I'm going to Toya's house, its Braxton's birthday," he said.

He licked his lips and took the palm of his hand to smooth down the lower part of his face. It was as if he knew I found it sexy.

The strangest thing for me, being twenty-seven years old, was being this mentally intimate with a man I never had sex with. Racing to a safe place in my thoughts, I was ready to talk about what we needed to take serious and to know if we can survive this test.

"Tony, I need you to stay in tonight, so we can talk about moving forward," I said.

Yes, despite the fact he never told me something everyone else knew; I was willing to make it work. My love was in charge and I was ready to shine a light on HIV and get a better understanding of how to love through his circumstances.

The topic of HIV was born and became common conversation between us. He wasn't afraid to talk about it with me and he helped me understand how to help him stay healthy.

"When a relationship changes the vision of your life, you no longer worry about the past, yet you focus on the breakthrough that is about to consume your struggles, that got you to where you are. The truth is...can you handle a breakthrough?"

—Joyful Soul

5 SECOND PROPOSAL

After me accepting the sentence and understanding the magnitude of this endorsement, a light began to shine in my soul. The following days carried so much weight to the knowledge I was seeking about the understanding of HIV.

I knew Tony and Magic Johnson had so much in common. The difference between the two was Mr. Johnson had financial means to support his treatment and Tony became an experimental specimen for them to research his condition at a prominent hospital in Winston-Salem, North Carolina. I was offended because he was being a guinea pig; for free!

Tony helped me understand the most important factor was he was healthy. I had all of the anger I felt he should have had even though we had not been sexual. Well, besides kissing and him performing oral on me.

Despite going through this since the early 80's and his near-death experience, he was so positive about our future. My love carried the weight of his pain, which began before I was ever born. We had much more to learn in order to go forward but it didn't stop Tony from lying next to me while watching a movie nor to propose again.

Tony reached into the nightstand drawer; where I knew he put that tainted ring. He gets down on both knees right when Tamika and Jacob enter the room. I looked at him with disgust on my face.

See, I had forgiven Tony but the ring was a symbolic link between deception and betrayal of my love. He looked into my eyes with the ring held open, while Jacob holds a sign that says YES, and Tamika holds a sign that says, MAYBE LATER.

"Shannon, I love you. I promise I will never bring a bridge between our relationship again. Will you be my wife?" Tears were flowing heavy down his face, "Please, Shannon, I need you."

"Tony, my love for you goes deeper than HIV. It is truly unconditional. Yes, I will marry you, but not with *that* ring."

As I watched our children, standing in the doorway, they were hugging one another and the bond between them became something we couldn't break up. Knowing the love they wanted was to be whole. It was amazing to me because at the time Tony and I were kissing, I was mentally focused on our children. They carried a burden of emptiness that was released with my 'yes'. I saw an angel wrapping around our family that was built with our love.

I didn't want the ring that held that level of pain, so I asked him to buy me any other ring. He ended up getting one from Amazon which was perfect because I am not materialistic. We chose to get married on my nephew's birthday because it was the day I realized my purpose of being a mother.

6 WEDDING

The days leading up to May 13, 2013, were hectic and very intense because my mom, stepdad, and sister, all still wanted to kill him. I had so much to do and so little time but I knew I was going to marry Tony, with or without the blessings of my family.

One thing I didn't think about was my son's biological father, Keith. He was my first love and nothing came between what we had until I made a public Facebook post announcing I was choosing Tony over him. Yet a part of my body still yearned for the passion to give my body to Keith but we agreed to stay away from each other. Even though our love was automatically generated, his desire to conceive children all over the state of North Carolina became a damaging factor to a successful relationship.

I had chosen a simple dress. My colors were silver, teal, and purple or eggplant. After work, I did everything for the wedding; getting measurements and finding the perfect suits for Jacob and for Tony. I loved this type of stuff. The joy I had was intense and the love he filled me with made loving him easy.

One night after getting home from a fitting, I told Tony when we got married and consummated our marriage, I would like to have another child. I didn't think he took me too seriously so I went to the doctor the next day to talk about our chances of having a child without HIV.

7 BABY FEVER

"Ms. Smith!" The nurse said as she came into the lobby area.

I walked back through the door with her and listened to her talk while my mind was on being with Tony and having another child. I was in a daze for a while until the doctor walked in.

"Hey, Ms. Smith, how are you feeling?" He questioned me with a concerned look.

"I am doing very well Doc. The initial shock is over and we have decided to stay together. The wedding is next Monday," I responded.

"I am glad you are okay now. Your test results are negative; so what brings you in here today?" Dr. B asked.

"I wanted to find out the options for Tony and me to have a child without the baby, nor me, catching HIV?" I asked.

"Shannon, I am going to be real with you," Dr. B responded. The process to complete a procedure like that would cost a lot of money because it's not covered by insurance. It's called the sperm washing process; where the HIV elements are extracted from the sperm and then inserted into you."

"How much is a lot because I want more children?" I said excitingly.

"To start the process, it would cost $20,000," he said.

I looked at him, "There is no way in hell. I don't wanted a child that bad."

When I got home, I called Tony and told him to come downstairs to let him know what the doctor said. I was crying; I didn't want to have HIV and I didn't want to be with anyone else either.

We talked about the option of adopting a child after we get married and found a house. He was okay with this decision but I was still a little skeptical because I enjoy the art of giving birth.

I had so many random thoughts run through my head like asking Tony for permission to have sex with Keith just once. I knew he was a certified impregnation machine but then I thought about Tony going crazy on me and the way my soul is; I love life and had no desire to die early.

Knowing the love for children that

drove deep within me, I had to suppress the feelings and focus on being Mrs. Tony Little. I was secure with Tony, our faith and trust grew daily and I had some of my family in my corner.

The week of the wedding I wanted everything to be perfect. I hired my mother's oldest sister, Aunt Flo; this woman could do anything she put her mind to. She was in Florence, South Carolina; therefore, I had to take a day off work to pick her up. I needed her to make my bouquet and the accent flowers for Jacob and Tony.

The marriage license was purchased and in Tony's hands. I think he kept it because he thought I was having second thoughts. However, I yearned for more children. My grandmother had eighteen and being a mother helped heal me in a way I didn't understand.

May 12, 2013, the day before I was going to marry this handsome fifty-six year old man at my ripe age of twenty-seven, my Aunt Flo still did not know about what happened at my surprise birthday party. However, what she did know was my mom still didn't like him. Naturally, she thought it was his age.

I had forgiven Tony and I wanted my mom to at least talk to him face to face. It was Mother's Day, the only gift I wanted, was for them to talk. I told this to Tony and he was willing to; I just had to get my mother, Cookie, to agree. Cookie is one stubborn woman; however, when it came to this, she agreed reluctantly.

It was about 11 am when my mom knocked on the door of my apartment. Immediately, I explained the rules, yes rules, because my mom will curse you and hit you, it was Mother's Day, I didn't want those problems. I explained to Tony and my mom, the importance of both of them in my life and made it clear there was to be no cursing, no hitting, or disrespect. They both agreed. Tony wasn't who I had to worry about.

After a few hours of talking, the white flag was flying high and there was a peaceful place between them. I so was overjoyed I asked Tony if he cared if we did it today, Mother's Day, at the Magistrate's office. Tony was nervous and excited at the same time and so was I.

I felt like I wanted to choke anyone who didn't come dressed right. Even though I was getting married earlier than we planned, nothing mattered but him and I. Saying I do was the most beautiful thing in the world when I looked at his smile and heard our children and family give us so much praise. Aunt Flo captured my view of the perfect bouquet. Her creation melted my heart; most of all, she was there to witness our love.

Going back to my apartment as his wife, nothing changed because he was always downstairs anyway. The consummation of our marriage was so beautiful. Tony purchased me a beautiful pure white gown, which I put on in the bathroom. I walked back into the room. The lights were turned off, lighted candles filled my bedroom, a fruit tray was on the bed, real rose petals led a pathway to the bed, and at the end of the petals; he was on his knees.

I could only think this man is going to make me fall in love with him again the closer I got to him. I ended at the petals and stood in front of him. He asked me to kneel down, I did, and he began to pray. For two and a half years, I had never seen, heard, or even knew he could pray.

After praying he indulged in the fruits of the labor which he planted. The pulsing feeling from the throbbing of his manhood made my body quiver with a deep desire. Sex with my husband was worth the wait and I became the happiest woman alive.

The next morning was the process of changing my last name. There were many things we already had in place and didn't want to change too much. We already agreed to move in together when we purchased our own home. I was glad for that because he was able to help his daughter.

She was out of work due to having to go to her appointments. Her boyfriend, who was not HIV positive, decided to stay with her. He was younger than her but he supported her as much as possible and never made her feel less than she was. We four were experiencing some of the purest levels of love given to mankind. We were always there for each other when any level of doubt arose. Yet, I was still fighting this baby battle.

My husband was taking every precaution to minimize my chance of ever transmitting HIV. We used toys, vibrators, role play, and oral indulgence. Tony never allowed me to perform oral on him which I understood.

I was being nosey and found out the same doctors who have been treating his HIV also suppressed his ability to climax. Before reading the documents I would have called anyone a liar. Yet, here I was with tears in my eyes.

We had been married for two months, and I was ovulating. I wanted to try and conceive a child. My coworker gave me a prescription that would counteract with the medicine he was taking. I told him it was an enhancer, that night, the passion was intense and mind-blowing. Even with the sex being mind-blowing as it was, Tony still didn't climax. He faked it! Yes, men can fake a climax.

8 AFFAIR

The next day, July 17, 2013, I was disappointed and frustrated. He could tell when he dropped me off at work. One thing about Tony was that he truly took care of me. I did not need to drive much since we did everything together. I arrived to work as usual and organized my workload.

Around 11 am, I got a call from Keith. He wanted me to come by his office which was a couple of blocks from my job, to help with a system he used for his security business. We talked on the phone and I told him about how my marriage was going and about me wanting another child.

He said in a joking manner, "I can fix that problem."

Part of me knew he wasn't joking at all. Keith was the type who wanted me all to himself while he was for everyone else. I'm sure you know the type.

"I know you can, but I love my husband, and you could never be who he is to me. I don't mind helping you with your business," I responded sarcastically.

It was true; everything within me loved that man but I just opened a door for him to come in. He knew I struggled with Tony not wanting to get me pregnant because of the risk of HIV. Keith knew much more than he should have known from a married woman. I felt guilty pouring our business out to anyone, but my heart just needed to cry a little. Word of advice: cry yourself to sleep, not in someone else's arms.

I was hesitant because whenever I was with Keith, it was never just business. In the back of my head, I knew it was going to get sexual. I went anyway and it was magical. I rushed back to work, I had to get myself together before Tony came to get me.

For the next week and a half Tony and I prepared for our wedding reception. There wasn't anything traditional about the way we wanted to do things but we were happy because we had our family and our children.

We found our dream home, more like Tony's dream home; I couldn't stand the steps. It was a great time for us to transition to our own home and Tony wanted to adopt Jacob.

Our life was coming together. I didn't have to think about the mistake I made with Keith. We had plans with the realtor to close on the house on August 9.

9 RECEPTION

On August 3, 2013, the day of the reception was amazing. Our families came, my had mom catered, and my mentor blessed Tony and I. After an exceptional reception I went home to see if my cycle had started. It hadn't. My monthly cycle had always been consistent since I was sixteen yet this month, it was a no-show.

While Tony and I relaxed on the couch, I got the notion to get up and test myself. I had a pregnancy test under my bathroom sink. My palms were sweaty, my head throbbed as the minutes passed, and when I looked at the test...I was pregnant. Holy crap, had we not been through enough?

I had to keep my composure as I walked back in the living room. Tony was reviewing the video from our wedding day on his iPad. I sat down next to him, looked him in his eyes and said that I was pregnant. The anger he had in his eyes before he spoke, scared me so much. I started to stand up and he grabbed my arm.

Tears rolled down my face as I was half stood up while Tony held my hand. I couldn't imagine what was going to happen next.

"What do you mean...you're pregnant?" Tony asked.

"When I was at work, the day we fought, Keith called me—" I started.

Before I could finish Tony jumped in and screamed, "I'M DONE, WE

ARE OVER! I'M NOT GOING TO HAVE PEOPLE LOOKING AT ME LIKE SOME F*****G SUCKA!"

The pain in the pit of my stomach hurt so bad. I wanted to erase my life from his and wave a wand to make him believe we could make it work. I turned my back to head towards the bedroom door then suddenly; the crash of the iPad was the next sound I heard. Tony walked out of my apartment and upstairs to the apartment he still shared with his daughter.

On his way out the door he said, "You wanted your baby? Now you have it, and the n***a who gave it to you."

I felt nothing, there were no more tears. The reality of it all became so real. I was faced with my husband telling my secret to anyone out of anger and the humiliation of having my family believe I could be carrying a child with HIV.

I called Tony to remind him of all the life plans we made and about closing on our house soon but I was greeted by the voicemail. I left multiple messages and finally, my last message was, "No child is worth losing the man I love. I feel a part of my heart is torn and saying sorry won't cut it, so I will make an appointment with the abortion clinic and remove this situation."

1:52 am, Tony called and said, "I got all of your messages. I wasn't ignoring you. I left my phone at home while I went with the boys. I was mad but it doesn't change my love for you and our family. And don't you ever think about having an abortion. Shan, you hear me?"

"Yes," I replied.

"Well okay, get yourself some sleep

and I will wake you up in the morning," he said slurring his word.

I began praying because at that time, going back to sleep, was not something I could accomplished. I was never able to experience the purity of grace and forgiveness by a physical being up until that point. I thanked the Most High and asked him for forgiveness as tears flowed, my nose stopped up, and my head throbbed. The affects of my praise, aided in my ability to fall asleep in peace.

Waking up to the smell of breakfast startled me, not because it was breakfast but mainly due to him sobering up so fast. I started to get up out of bed and Tony told me to lie down and stay in bed; I did.

He came into the room with my breakfast on a tray, flowers, and he said, "I want you to make sure our child eats well." Tony sat next to me with the deepest level of concern on his face.

I said, "Just ask me what's on your mind."

Tony questioned, "Was there any other time and is there anyone else?"

I was happy to tell him, "Yes, Tony that was the only time and there was no one else."

The excitement for me to live in my truth was so powerful. I felt the burden of guilt lift away as I was eating the breakfast he prepared. Then something I remembered made me pause and I had to be sure he was ready to face this with me.

"Tony, are you okay with going forward with our marriage and this child?" I asked with curiosity.

"Yes, I'm sure. If anyone asks it is my child and that is that. I don't want to talk about this anymore. Let's move past this," the words of a confident and dominant Tony.

I knew then my heart was sold and I would be devoted to loving and appreciating him for the rest of our lives together. He had a stronghold on my love, loyalty, faith, and my commitment. There was something about the man that was familiar and unfamiliar at the same time. It was like a love you pray for when you're a lost soul.

My heart was changing. The molecules in my brain began to process love a little differently. I found myself in my closet crying and telling God, "Thank you for blessing me any way." I was in a place of devotion and security. My love for Tony grew more and more as we went through the pregnancy together.

The bondage I thought held me down was loosened by an act of true love. The kind of love that keeps you up late at night writing love letters and poems until you fall asleep. Something about the connection between Tony and I had reactivated that kiddie love. My mind and soul were in a new place and I was ready to live in my forever's arms.

Keith knew the decision Tony and I made; he didn't care at all, and we didn't try to make him care. I felt a sense of release knowing we had a secret and a bond which gave us more power and no one could take that away from us.

10 HOME SWEET, HOME

Our journey, looking for our home during this process, had finally come to an end. Tony loved everything about the house. I could not stand the three levels, equaling a lot of stairs, knowing my left knee would give out. I commonly referred to the house as Tony's dream home even though we used the VA Home Loan and my credit being to buy it.

The home was everything he wanted; his love for it was like watching a secret love affair. It brought me joy to see him happy after having to go through so much in life before me, and with me. Tony did everything in the home, which also made buying the home so much easier.

It was August 9, 2013, our closing day for Tony's dream home. I felt like I was signing my soul to the devil as Tony signed his five or so documents then proceeded to watch me. The process of signing hurt my mind and my hand. I was sleepy when it was over because I didn't think we would see daylight. Being in the attorney's office for the amount of time increased my anxiety of wanting a home.

Finally, it was over and Tony was happy he had his keys. I was nonchalant about it the entire time. Then when I thought about it, this was his dream, the process had very little to do with me, I was a gateway. When it came to this mindset, I had made peace with a lot of my past experiences and knew God had blessed me to help meet the needs of others.

A part of Tony and my healing was understanding we were going to have to let God lead our lives. I had to learn to allow Tony to be the husband God had for me and he was all of that and more. Moving into our new home, I did no heavy lifting, Tony wasn't going for that. He wanted to protect his wife and unborn child at all costs. Tony and one of his cousins unloaded all of our belongings into the home; while I called the cable man for standard hookups and Duke Energy to transfer our lights.

The arrangements we had in place worked great towards accomplishing things, using our strong suits. The next day, it was work as usual for me. It was an ordinary day until Tony picked me up. When I got in the car, he smelt like he had been cooking. This was strange for today because he said he was going to unpack while I was working. While we were on our way home I stared at him weird the entire time. I was ready to fuss.

I walked in the front door and the strong aroma of fresh dinner welcomed me warmly. I looked around; I could not believe my husband had the three-level home completely put together; no boxes left in sight. This man took my love to a new level. The dedication and commitment he was showing, to be the best husband he could've been.

The next several months, our life was full of social gatherings, prenatal appointments, and taking Jacob on various adventures.

11 MORNING SICKNESS

Being pregnant meant a lot of my habits had to change. I had to stop drinking, going to clubs, and most of all, I had to really be committed to being devoted to my marriage. The giving up of certain things became natural; however, I needed to stop taking an antidepressant. I was diagnosed with depression after an abusive relationship in 2009.

This relationship helped me in a multitude of ways when it came to understanding the level of manipulation within the world. Depression wasn't the only thing I had to battle during this pregnancy, although the condition had its share of damages nonetheless.

When I called my Veteran Health Administration Mental Health doctor, they informed me to stop taking my antidepressant right away. I was not too sure about this idea but I wanted to do what was best for my unborn child. I learned very quickly I had an addiction.

I started to wake up with chills after a week of stopping my citalopram. I knew something was wrong with me. Tony held me close every night to show me I was safe. I was out of work for a week and didn't care about the magnitude this absence would have on my career. Nothing mattered. Tony told me to go to the emergency room at the VAMC and they would have to do something. I agreed, this issue was not pleasant and I needed them to make things better.

One night after church I lost my ability to see; literally blind. I told Tony about the blindness and he said, "Baby, I know you are trying to tough this out but it's time to go to an outside doctor." I understood exactly where he was coming from but I didn't like the long wait times and hated being told, "There is nothing we can do." Tony's concern for my safety grew greatly.

It had been a week and a half without me being able to eat and I drank the bare minimum. Tony was tired of asking for my consent and took me to Forsyth Medical Center. I waited in the wheelchair dizzy, confused, and drained from the lack of any nutrients. Tony talked to the nurse about my condition. I don't know what he said, but I heard a nurse inform him, "Taking a pregnant woman off an antidepressant, cold turkey, can kill the fetus."

Her words brought tears to my eyes and I could not explain why I was crying. I was just so lost on what to do next. Tony was my hero; the feeling of blindness led me to rely solely on his leadership. I didn't know it at the time but God blinded me to shut me down from wanting to be in control of everything.

The nursing staff took me immediately the back and put me on three different machines. They put an IV in me, hooked me to the machine in order to monitor the baby's heart rate, and a machine to administer medicine to would relieve my feeling. Within the hour, I was feeling better.

Four nurses came in to check on

me and to thank Tony for bringing me in. I thought God was punishing me for cheating on my husband. Nothing compared to going through this horrific event with the love of my life. I knew he had me and my best interest at heart. Doctors will never compare to the actions of the nurses who shadow under them. I couldn't have had a better team to set me free from that type of pain.

I learn that being taken off an antidepressant would give you the same effect as an addict withdrawing from drugs. I knew cheating would never be an option in my life and I knew I would stay true to love, no matter the circumstance.

12 NEW YEAR'S RESOLUTION

For a new year's resolution, I set a challenge for Tony to stop smoking and drinking. We were expecting our baby girl in April and I wanted to be prepared. Tony accepted my challenge and that's when he started to feel levels of pain that would change our life forever.

Our home was a place of comfort but Tony wasn't comfortable by a long shot. I started to notice he would forget things and he was in constant pain, so I told him that he could start smoking again if he felt as that would help him not feel pain.

Tony went his annual check-up in early January 2014 and I was adamant about him letting his doctors know about his pain. He told the doctors about everything that was bothering him and they ran numerous test. At home, Tony continued to be in pain, but his care of the family and home never went down. I was blessed to have a man devoted to his family and his craft, for it to not affect his ability to do what he was born to do.

January 27, 2014, Tony and I were called in by his infectious disease doctor, which was a little scary. I thought the manifestation of AIDS was taking over but that was not the news we were about to hear. Being called into the office that Monday was a scare.

The social worker for infectious

disease patients came into the small patient room and began to ask us about will preparation and funeral costs. I knew what it meant and so did Tony, and for some weird reason, he didn't look as surprised as I did. As the social worker exited the room, he told us that the doctor would provide us with more details.

Tony and I were in a great place spiritually and we knew this day would come. Thirty-five minutes later, two doctors entered the room to inform us that Tony had lesions on his lung, liver, and bone. In my heart, I believed he could be healed but my mind knew this was our last days.

"Doctor, is there a way you can check his brain activity as well because he has been forgetting a lot as of late?" I asked the doctor sitting down closest to me.

"Yes, we can do an MRI. When is

the best day for you?" he asked.

"How about February 6, 2014, as early as possible?" I asked. Tony sat there with minimum response to the situation and I hugged him. "We got this, no matter what." Nothing could prepare my heart for the series of events to come next.

13 THE FALL

February 6, 2014, we woke super early to attend the MRI, drop Jacob off, and I was going to go to work. I believe we started our morning about 6 am so we would be able to get everything done in time. McDonald's was our first stop for breakfast, and this time, I needed to drive due to Tony struggling with his vision. The task of driving was difficult because I was pregnant in a little Toyota Corolla and I suffered with morning sickness or with withdrawal symptoms my entire pregnancy.

After the stop for our breakfast, we arrived at the MRI building for the test to be conducted. As we got out of the car, with food in all of our hands, Tony begins to call my name.

"Yes, honey what's wrong?" I asked with deep concern.

"Shan, I can't walk, my legs won't move!" he exclaimed.

"Okay, baby hold on. Let me put this down and I will help you."

My heart and soul only thought about holding my 6'1 husband and getting him into the office. Even though I was eight months pregnant at the time; my stomach nor its size mattered. Seeing my husband almost collapse, I wrapped my arms around him. The heavier he became the lower I kneeled to help him to the ground safely.

Pitch black and no traffic in sight, I asked God to bless me with a child of obedience. I looked Jacob in the face, who was three years old at the time, and said, "I want you to go across the street and get help, so listen carefully. Go to the end of this parking lot and look both ways before you cross the street. Go to the class door and tell the person at the desk that your Daddy is at the MRI building and has fallen. They needed to bring a stretcher. If no one is there, yell at the top of your lungs for HELP."

Jacob was full of tears but said, "Yes, ma'am, I will go get us help."

He did exactly that. Soon there were multiple emergency responders there with us within seconds of Jacob leaving. During the time of me hearing them come to our aid, I also heard Tony make a gurgling sound.

I turned him on his side and a stream of saliva began to pour out. I rubbed his back and told him help was on the way. When help arrived it was an intense moment for me. The responders were trying to get me to get checked out as they were trying to figure out what happened to Tony. I was determined to stay by his side and nothing or no one could change what I was feeling.

The hospital ran numerous tests and found out that Tony had lesions on his brain near his spinal gateway which sends the fluid to his spine to aid in his motor skills. The pain of this news traveled through my body and I collapsed. The emergency aid rushed to my side and assisted me coming to grips with the magnitude of the news.

Tony was later transferred to the oncology floor of the hospital. During this time of the year, we started to experience a great deal of snow which delayed a lot of the services he would have gotten faster. I stayed at the hospital with my husband and ensured his comfort level was at the utmost. As his wife, my job to protect him became evident and I wanted to do that at all cost.

14 DIAGNOSIS AND DEVOTION

On February 13, 2014, several doctors came in to assess Tony and to determine what could be done. They also told us the name of the condition was, Stage 4 adencarcinoma lung cancer. It had metastasized to his brain, lung, liver, and bone.

A couple days later, my best friend, my lover, my husband wanted to go home and it gave me much joy to have him holding onto my arms. When we got home, we talked so much about how to handle the kids, about him wanting me to re-marry before he leaves and about never forgetting what we shared. The doctors requested that he see the radiologist to reduce the lesions on his brain. I took him to each appointment; the last one being February 26, 2014.

The next morning we woke up and my husband was no longer my himself. He accused me of withholding his medicine and holding him hostage. I knew his mind was no longer able to function on a suitable level. I called hospice in to assist me. I still felt this was my responsibility, yet I recognized when I would be unable to do this alone. Every day for the next week, I was by his side, praying for peace, healing, and understanding.

I lay next to Tony, slept with him, and bathed him even though his motor skills were gone. Nothing took me away from giving Tony my all in his last days. On March 7, 2014, the hospice nurse called me in our bedroom. I was in the living room talking on the phone with my aunt. She told me Tony's breathing was getting deeper. I walked into the room and held his hand as he took his last breath.

The nurse announced his death at 11:10 am; I called Jacob, who was with my mom at the time; to let him know his dad had passed away. My parents came shortly.

Jacob walked in the door and said, "Mami, don't cry, dad isn't in pain anymore. I'm going to go kiss him and tell him goodbye."

Before I could respond, Jacob was in the room with his father lying in the bed. Jacob returned to the living room with no tears and he showed me the power of loving with a pure heart.

Tony changed our lives and gave us something we never had. The power of his story helped me to be a better woman, mother, and friend. He had a condition that could have taken him out but it took more than the HIV to bring him down. He encouraged my will to love and tell our story, so others will know they can find hope, love, and strength.

STAY CURRENT

Recent Article on HIV by NAM Publications

HIV update - 22nd November 2017

You may have an undetectable viral load, but your partner may still need PrEP or PEP.

New HIV infections among the HIV-negative gay men in the PARTNER study, due to sex with partners outside the main relationship, was high, a recent conference heard.

PARTNER made headlines by demonstrating that there were no transmissions from an HIV positive partner who was on antiretroviral therapy and virally suppressed in almost 60,000 acts of condomless sex.

These data allowed the researchers to establish the maximum possible likelihood of transmission, and to announce that, most likely, the chance of an HIV positive partner with a fully suppressed viral load of below 200 copies/ml passing on HIV was zero. PARTNER provides crucial evidence for the U=U (Undetectable = Untransmittable) campaign.

However, there were HIV infections in PARTNER: eleven of them by 2016, ten in gay men. In all cases, however, phylogenetic testing showed that the infecting virus came from someone other than the primary partner.

Each year, 2% of HIV-negative gay male partners acquired HIV. Looking only at those men who reported having condomless anal sex with non-primary partners, each year 7% acquired HIV.

In short, men whose main partner is undetectable are not safe from HIV if they are also having condomless sex with other people. In this situation, it would make sense for the HIV-negative man to use post-exposure prophylaxis (PEP) or pre-exposure prophylaxis (PrEP).

But very few of those taking part in the PARTNER study did so, resulting in these high levels of infection.

HPV and anal cancer

HPV (human papillomavirus) is a sexually transmitted virus that causes genital warts, and in some forms, leads to the development of cervical, anal, mouth and throat cancers.

Anal cancer, rare in the general population, is becoming more common in people living with HIV, especially men who have sex with men.

The European AIDS Clinical Society has strengthened its advice on vaccination against HPV. All people living with HIV under the age of 26 and all gay men living with HIV under the age of 40 should be vaccinated, it says.

These recommendations are in line with the guidance of the British HIV Association (BHIVA).

The reason why these guidelines include upper age limits is that the older you are, the more likely it is that you have already been exposed to several types of HPV, making the vaccine less effective. The younger you are, the more likely you are to benefit from vaccination.

Recently, Dutch clinicians reported on their experience of screening gay men living with HIV for pre-cancerous anal lesions. This is not the same as anal cancer, but having these pre-cancerous cell changes is associated with a small risk of developing cancer in the future. The lesions might go away on their own, but in case they don't, many doctors would recommend treatment.

Of just under 1700 men who were screened, they found that 30% had high-grade lesions. Given this high rate, the clinicians believe that screening all gay men living with HIV would be a good idea.

Nonetheless, screening for precancerous anal cell changes in people who don't have symptoms is not currently recommended in guidelines. This is because we don't yet know whether the available treatments are good enough to make screening worthwhile in people who haven't got symptoms. The treatments can be uncomfortable, have side-effects and don't always stop high-grade lesions from recurring. It could be worrying to find out that you have pre-cancerous lesions, but if you didn't know you had them, it's possible that they would go away on their own or cause you no harm.

On the other hand, some experts believe that finding and treating high-grade lesions promptly will prevent cases of anal cancer that would be much harder to treat later on, so they think it is worth getting tested regularly.

These doctors also point to high rates of anal cancer in gay men living with HIV, for example a recent analysis from Austria – in men under 50 years, 8 in 1000 had ever had anal cancer; in men over 50 years, 26 in 1000 had ever had it. As the risk of cancer increases the older we get and more people with HIV are going to live longer in future years, these rates could increase further as time goes on.

Does U=U apply to breastfeeding?

Taking effective HIV treatment and having an undetectable viral load massively reduces the risk of onward transmission during breastfeeding, but it does not appear that the risk is zero, a leading paediatrician from St Mary's Hospital, London said last week. Dr. Hermione Lyall said that she often needed to advise women who were doing well on HIV treatment, with an undetectable viral load, who wished to breastfeed.

Studies from African countries suggest that for women with HIV taking treatment (not necessarily undetectable), around 1 to 2 in 100 may pass on HIV to their baby. More reassuringly, a recent Tanzanian study found that among 177 mothers, there were no transmissions from mothers with undetectable viral loads. This suggests that there is a very low risk of breastfeeding transmission when viral load is suppressed, but these are not enough data to say that the statement "undetectable=untransmittable" (U=U) applies to breastfeeding as well as to sexual transmission.

Dr. Lyall says that women with HIV should be advised that formula feeding has a zero risk of HIV transmission and is the safest thing to do. Nonetheless, some women will choose to breastfeed and healthcare professionals should support them to do so as safely as possible.

Mothers should be advised that having an undetectable viral load, taking all their doses of their treatment and limiting the duration of breastfeeding will help lower the risk of passing HIV on. They should attend monthly check-ups with their clinical teams.

Dr. Lyall also presented three key safety points that women should remember while they breastfeed:

No virus:
Only breastfeed if your HIV is undetectable.

Happy tums:
Only breastfeed if both you and your baby are free from tummy problems.

Healthy breasts for mums:
Only breastfeed if your breasts and nipples are healthy with no signs of injury or infection.

Healthcare workers living with HIV

Nurses and other healthcare workers who are living with HIV have mixed reactions when they mention their HIV status to colleagues, according to a small Dutch study. Some healthcare workers disclosed because they were confident they would have a positive reaction or because concealment was stressful. Very often, those disclosed to saw the participant's HIV status as a non-issue, as one interviewee explained:

"In the beginning, it was talked about and thought about a lot but that was, at a given moment, gone and nobody gave it anymore thought."

Other interviewees concealed because they did not believe that disclosure was relevant or necessary. Some people did not discuss their HIV status because they expected negative reactions or stigma, often because they had previously experienced this themselves or had seen it occur in relation to other people.

"I'm not going to tell them anymore because I'm, yeah, I'm scared of how my colleagues will react. And where does this come from? It comes from, for example, the fact that whenever a patient is admitted and he has HIV, then they immediately say, 'You need to be careful, eh? He has HIV so be extra careful'."

The researchers say that it's important to emphasize that disclosure is a choice. Before disclosing at work, people should think carefully about their motivations for disclosure and the potential reactions they might have. The authors comment that while disclosure can be a good idea if it results in social support or less stress, it may sometimes be better to conceal at work, especially when the risks are great and social support is available elsewhere.

Heart disease and kidney disease

Cardiovascular disease (angina, heart failure, stroke, blocked arteries etc) goes hand in hand with chronic kidney disease, according to an analysis of over 27,000 people living with HIV.

People who were assessed as being at high risk of cardiovascular disease were also more likely to go on to have kidney disease. Similarly, being at high risk of kidney disease increased people's risk of having cardiovascular disease. Rates of subsequent disease were especially high in people who had been assessed as being at risk of both.

The researchers say that doctors should assess the risk of these conditions together. They should also focus on encouraging people with HIV to make lifestyle changes which lower the risk of both conditions – eat a healthy, balanced diet; exercise regularly; lose weight if you're overweight; don't smoke; and limit your intake of drugs and alcohol.

Misuse of the term 'stigma' continues to control the behaviors of people living with HIV. It is all too common to blame this monster in the dark, a beast lurking on the streets than it is to blame our own family and friends, the people we love for their fear or ignorance. And we also need to stop telling people living with HIV that they will be stigmatized.

NAM's information is intended to support, rather than replace, consultation with a healthcare professional. Talk to your doctor or another member of your healthcare team for advice tailored to your situation.

NAM Publications
Registered office:
Acorn House, 314-320
Gray's Inn Road,
London, WC1X 8DP
Company limited by guarantee. Registered in England & Wales, number: 2707596
Registered charity, number: 1011220
© NAM Publications, 2017.
All rights reserved.

www.ingramcontent.com/pod-product-compliance
Lightning Source LLC
Chambersburg PA
CBHW070312230526
45470CB00002B/834